Scriptures

&

Prayers For

Pregnant Women

Tatang D. Hubert R.

1

All scriptures used in this book are taken from the King James Version of the Holy Bible unless otherwise stated.

Scriptures & Prayers For Pregnant Women

ISBN-13: 978-1530615940

ISBN-10: 1530615941

3

Lo, children *are* an heritage of the LORD: *and* the fruit of the womb *is his* reward.

As arrows *are* in the hand of a mighty man; so *are* children of the youth.

Happy *is* the man that hath his quiver full of them: they shall not be ashamed, but they shall speak with the enemies in the gate, Ps 127:3-5.

Blessed *is* every one that feareth the LORD; that walketh in his ways.

For thou shalt eat the labour of thine hands: happy *shalt* thou *be,* and *it shall be* well with thee.

Thy wife *shall be* as a fruitful vine by the sides of thine house: thy children like olive plants round about thy table.

Behold, that thus shall the man be blessed that feareth the LORD.

The LORD shall bless thee out of Zion: and thou shalt see the good of Jerusalem all the days of thy life. Yea, thou shalt see thy children's children, *and* peace upon Israel, **Ps 128:1-6**.

PRAYER DURING PREGNANCY

Place your hands on your belly before praying and repeat over and over until delivery. Often anoint your stomach with anointing oil before praying. If you have already decided the name of your child, which I advise you to do, call his/her name from time to time, and bless him.

[Children are a reward from the Lord, children are a blessing, and the blessing of God makes rich and happy, He adds no sorrow to it, according to Proverbs 10: 22. So I declare that my pregnancy is a blessing, my baby is a source of joy and happiness, and not of sorrow and pains. I will give birth to my baby without problems, even before labor comes. I will deliver my child through normal process. The God who gave me

this child is with me, and His Mighty Hand is upon me always will until delivery. It is written, "Before Zion was in labor, she gave birth; before she was in pain, she delivered a boy. Who has heard of such a thing? Who has seen such things? Can a land be born in one day or a nation be delivered in an instant? Yet as soon as Zion was in labor, she gave birth to her sons. "Will I bring a baby to the point of birth and not deliver [it]?" says the LORD; "or will I who deliver, close [the womb]?" says your God. Be glad for Jerusalem and rejoice over her, all who love her. Rejoice greatly with her, all who mourn over her", according to Isaiah 66:7-10 (HCSB). I am the woman the Bible is talking about. I declare that any weapon formed against me and my baby will have no effect, it shall not prosper. I decree by the

Holy Spirit, "Before I travailed, before I am in labor, I have brought forth my child." I declare and decree with insurance in the Powerful Name of Jesus Christ, before my pain came, I have given birth to my child. The word of God does not lie, God is committed to fulfill His word in my life. So I declare in the Precious Name of Jesus Christ, as soon as I am in labor, I, the daughter of Zion, give birth to my healthy son! The Lord is my shepherd, I will fear nothing. He is with me, so everything will be fine. Thank you Lord Jesus, for Your powerful Hand on my life now and forever. I surrender myself to you, because I know you cannot disappoint me.

O God, arise and act in my life. I give myself entirely to you this day, and I choose to follow you the rest of my life, and abandon the life of sin.

Lord Jesus, hear me and come to my rescue.
Today I have chosen you as my master and my
husband. Sanctify and cleanse me with Your
precious Blood, deliver me from the power of
Satan, demons and sin to serve the living God. I
receive the Holy Spirit into my life, to walk in the
truth and worship in spirit and in truth you.]

PRAYER FOR DIFFICULT OR UNSTABLE PREGNANCY

When having problems and difficulties with pregnancy read and meditate scriptures such as **Isaiah 66:7-10, Exodus 23: 25-26,** then declare the word of God to the womb, speak the word of God to the unborn child. Pray prayers such as suggested below all through the pregnancy period. Lay hands on the womb, anoint it with anointing oil if possible and pray:

[Children are a reward from the Lord, children are a blessing, and the blessing of God makes rich and happy, He adds no sorrow to it, according to **Proverbs 10: 22**. So I declare that my pregnancy is a blessing, my baby is a source of joy and happiness, and not of sorrow and pains. I will give birth to my

11

baby without problems, even before labor comes. I will deliver my child through normal process. The God who gave me this child is with me, and His Mighty Hand is upon me always will until delivery. It is written, **"Before Zion was in labor, she gave birth; before she was in pain, she delivered a boy. Who has heard of such a thing? Who has seen such things? Can a land be born in one day or a nation be delivered in an instant? Yet as soon as Zion was in labor, she gave birth to her sons. "Will I bring a baby to the point of birth and not deliver [it]?" says the LORD; "or will I who deliver, close [the womb]?" says your God. Be glad for Jerusalem and rejoice over her, all who love her. Rejoice greatly with her, all who mourn over her"**, accord to **Isaiah 66:7-10 (HCSB)**.

I am the woman the Bible is talking about. I declare

that any weapon formed against me and my baby will have no effect, it shall not prosper. I decree by the Holy Spirit, "Before I travailed, before I am in labor, I have brought forth my child." I declare and decree with insurance in the Powerful Name of Jesus Christ, before my pain came, I have given birth to my child. The word of God does not lie, God is committed to fulfill His word in my life. So I declare in the Precious Name of Jesus Christ, as soon as I am in labor, I, the daughter of Zion I give birth to my son! The Lord is my shepherd, I will fear nothing. He is with me, so everything will be fine. Thank you Lord Jesus, for Your powerful Hand on my life now and forever. I surrender myself to you, because I know you cannot disappoint me.

O God, arise and act in my life. I give myself entirely to you this day, and I choose to follow you the rest of my life, and abandon the life of sin. Lord Jesus, hear me and come to my rescue. Today I have chosen you as my master and my husband. Sanctify and cleanse me with Your precious Blood, deliver me from the power of Satan, demons and sin to serve the living God. I receive the Holy Spirit into my life, to walk in the truth and worship in spirit and in truth you].

NOW STAND FIRM IN THE LORD!

FINALLY, MY BRETHREN, BE
STRONG IN THE LORD, and in the power of his
might. Put on the whole armour of God, that ye
may be able to stand against the wiles of the devil.
For we wrestle not against flesh and blood, but
against principalities, against powers, against the
rulers of the darkness of this world, against
spiritual wickedness in high places. Wherefore
take unto you the whole armour of God, THAT
YE MAY BE ABLE TO WITHSTAND IN THE
EVIL DAY, AND HAVING DONE ALL, TO
STAND. STAND THEREFORE, having your

**loins girt about with truth, and having on the
breastplate of righteousness; And your feet shod
with the preparation of the gospel of peace;
Above all, taking the shield of faith, wherewith ye
shall be able to quench all the fiery darts of the
wicked. And take the helmet of salvation, and the
sword of the Spirit, which is the word of God:
Praying always with all prayer and supplication
in the Spirit, and watching thereunto with all
perseverance and supplication for all saints,**
Ephesians 6: 10-18.

Of you move out of Christ, you are gone.
Christ is your only security against satan and his

horrors.

Learn to resist sickness and all afflictions of the devil. Nothing settles in your life without your permission. The problem is neither with God, nor the devil. You are the problem. If you make your mind to live healthy, you can. To ride on over the devil and live a victorious and triumphant Christian life, you must locate a living and Spirit-filled church, and abide there. Do not follow religion, do not follow the church because someone has brought you there or because it is a family church, but because you are convicted God is there. Be there because you are taught God's word. I am not saying you should not follow your family to the same church, but be careful not to follow people in error and you know it. Seek God personally and have a relationship with Him out of love and sincerity.

Also, get your copy of our books **"DIVINE HEALING IS STILL POSSIBLE"**, and **"WHO IS A CHRISTIAN"**, by the same author, and you will greatly be blessed. Feel free also to contact us for help and counseling.

But most importantly, understand that God is not responsible of your mediocre living, and it is not holiness. Satan is your problem, if does anything in your life it is because you allow Him. Look at what happened in the Garden of Eden. When man fell, God knew very well how it happened. But he asked man, because satan was not supposed to operate. It was man's duty to put the devil where he belongs, and control the garden as God had charged him.

Your health, your marriage, your business, your finances, education, children, etc, are what constitute your garden, and it is your responsibility to determine what happens to it. I am talking to those in Christ.

In the garden, **"And the LORD God planted**

a garden eastward in Eden; and there he put the man whom he had formed... And the LORD God took the man, and put him into the Garden of Eden to DRESS it and to KEEP it" Genesis 2: 8; 15

To dress means to put it in order and in good shape. To KEEP it means to control and watch over. It was not satan that was given charge over the garden, but man. Now, look at what happened (Matthew 13: 24-28, 38-37);

Another parable put he forth unto them, saying, The kingdom of heaven is likened unto a

man which sowed GOOD SEED in his field: But WHILE MEN SLEPT, his enemy came and sowed tares among the wheat, and went his way. But when the blade was sprung up, and brought forth fruit, then appeared the tares also. So the servants of the householder came and said unto him, Sir, didst not thou sow good seed in thy field? from whence then hath it tares? He said unto them, An enemy hath done this...He answered and said unto them, HE THAT SOWETH THE GOOD SEED IS THE SON OF MAN ...The enemy that sowed them is the DEVIL".

If you sleep over your life, and health, be ready for tares. Now, when Christ came, He gave unto us what it takes to dominate and have the last say over our health, and entire life on earth;

Luke 10: 19 **Behold, I give unto you power to tread on serpents and scorpions, and over all the power of the enemy: and nothing shall by any means hurt you.**

That is why you are called to resist him; that is, to stop him from sowing tares in your life. Jesus will not come and resist him for you. Neither Mary, nor his angels will come and tread over his power for you, you have to.

ABOUT THE AUTHOR

HUBERT TATANG; is an ordained minister of Jesus Christ, a young missionary called by God and trained in China. He began fulltime missionary service in 2007, and has ever since been instrumental in the hands of God in the mission field in Africa, precisely in Cameroon and Nigeria.

Prince Hubert is a Tele and Radio evangelist, and teacher in seminar and conference Speaker. He is a teacher on marriage and healing.

His is a writer and author of several books including:

Morning Shower (a daily devotional),

Divine Healing Is Still Possible… Volume 1 & 2,

The Beauty and the Riches of Redemption (Vol. 1 & 2),

The Good Shepherd, Total Victory Over Sicknesses…

<u>**Contact the Author**</u>:

(+237) 679 71 62 90 - 694 07 51 32.

<u>princeofj@gmail.com</u>

www.ingramcontent.com/pod-product-compliance
Lightning Source LLC
Chambersburg PA
CBHW022341290526
45786CB00013B/2011